Harcourt

Health and Fitness

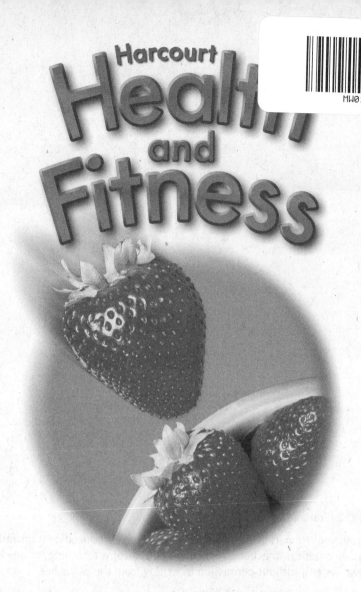

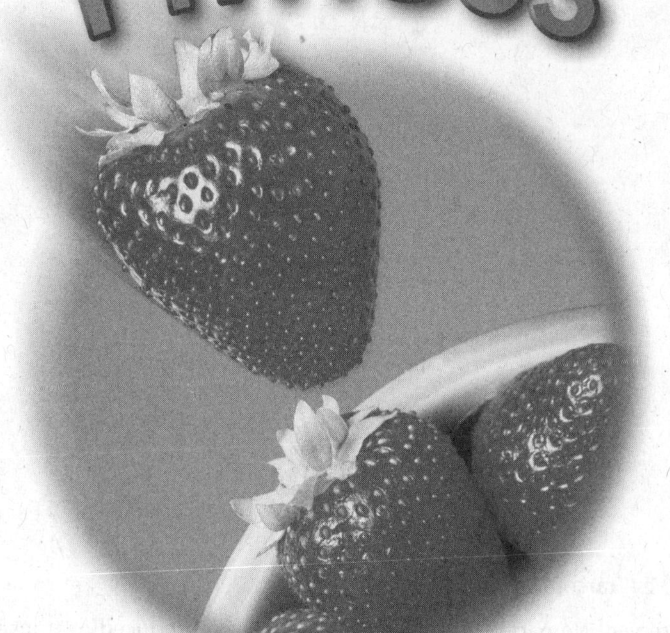

Activity Book

Grade 6

Harcourt
SCHOOL PUBLISHERS

Orlando • Austin • New York • San Diego • Toronto • London

Visit *The Learning Site!*
www.harcourtschool.com

Printed in the United States of America

ISBN 13: 978-0-15-355144-4
ISBN 10: 0-15-355144-5

5 6 7 8 9 10 073 15 14 13 12 11 10 09

Contents

CHAPTER 7

Controlling Disease

CHAPTER 8

Drugs and Health

CHAPTER 9

Tobacco and Alcohol

CHAPTER 10

Setting Goals

CHAPTER 11

Family and Responsibility

CHAPTER 12

Community Health

CHAPTER 1

Name ______________________________

Quick Study

Growth and Development

Directions

- Use lesson vocabulary in the Word Bank to complete each **Summary**.
- Read the directions provided to complete each **Lesson Details**.

Word Bank

abstinence	DNA	fetus	maturity	puberty
adolescence	embryo	genes	pituitary gland	sperm
circulatory system	endocrine system	excretory system	respiratory system	

Lesson 1 pp. 4–11

Summary Oxygen enters your body through your ______________________ and is carried to all parts of your body by your ______________________. The skin, kidneys, and bladder are parts of the ______________________, which removes waste.

Lesson Details Fill in the table to show how body systems work together.

This system	depends on this system	to
nervous		protect the brain and spinal cord
circulatory		exchange oxygen and carbon dioxide
digestive	muscular	
muscular	nervous	

Lesson 2 pp. 12–18

Summary It takes one ________________ to fertilize an ovum. The new cell grows and becomes an ________________. After the second month of development, the embryo is called a ________________. Chromosomes are made up of ________________. Genes are parts of ________________, the chemical code for inherited traits.

Name ______________________________

Lesson Details Number the following steps in order.

____ Major organs form in developing baby.	____ Cells divide to form embryo.	____ Developing baby begins to move.
____ Baby is born.	____ Ovum and sperm combine.	____ Lungs are capable of breathing.

Lesson 3 pp. 20–27

Summary The ________________ is one of the glands that make up the ________________. This gland causes the development of eggs and sperm in a process called ________________. This process happens during ________________.

Lesson Details Use page 23 to complete the graphic organizer.

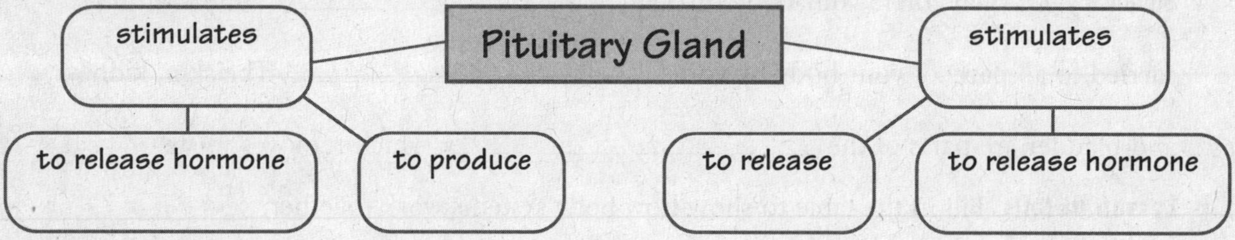

Lesson 4 pp. 28–31

Summary At the end of adolescence, you will reach a stage of life called ____________.

Lesson Details Describe the ways your attitudes will change during adolescence toward your family. ____

____

Lesson 5 pp. 34–36

Summary You can take care of your health by practicing ______________.

Lesson Details For each unhealthful behavior, write a healthful alternative.

Unhealthful Behavior	Healthful Alternative
Drinking alcohol when bored	________________
Smoking tobacco when stressed	________________
Spending the afternoon watching TV	________________

Name ______________________________

Focus Skill **Reading Skill**

Sequence

Blood Flow Through the Heart

The heart is a muscular organ that pumps blood through the blood vessels. It has four chambers, or spaces, that blood enters and leaves. The two upper chambers, called atria, receive the blood that is returning from the body and the lungs. The two lower chambers, called ventricles, pump out the blood to the body and the lungs.

Large veins carry blood from the body back to the heart. This blood is low in oxygen. It enters the heart's right atrium and then goes to the right ventricle. The right ventricle pumps the blood through a large artery to the lungs, where it picks up oxygen. Large veins carry this oxygen-rich blood to the heart's left atrium. The blood then goes to the left ventricle, which pumps it out through a large artery to all parts of the body.

Use the graphic organizer to draw arrows showing the sequence of blood flow through the heart. You may have arrows that cross. After you have completed the graphic organizer, explain why this statement is incorrect: "All arteries carry oxygen-rich blood, and all veins carry oxygen-poor blood."

____

____

____

____

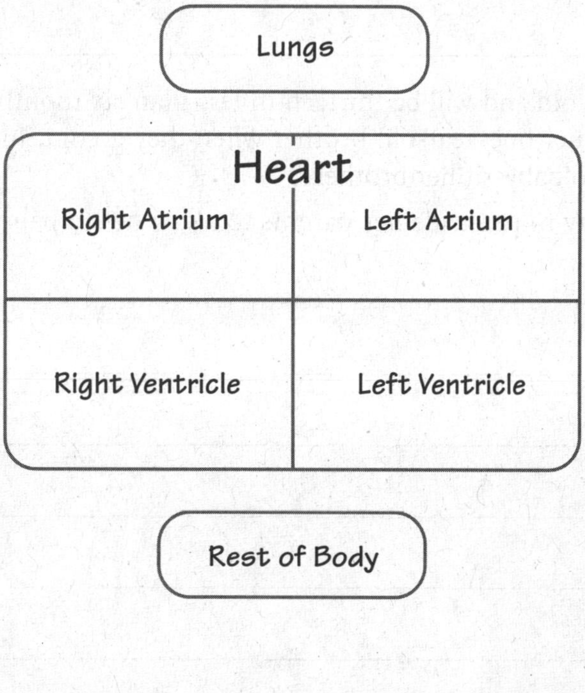

Name ______________________

Problem Solving

Life Skill

Communicate

Steps for Effective Communication

1. Understand your audience.
2. Give a clear message. Use "I" messages.
3. Listen carefully, and answer any questions.
4. Gather feedback.

Tell how these students would use the steps to communicate effectively.

A. Andy's friend Davis has started calling him "Stringbean" because Andy has recently grown taller but has not filled out yet. Andy doesn't like the nickname. One day he tells Davis, "I'm tired of your being disrespectful and mean." Davis responds, "You hurt my feelings. I don't want to be your friend anymore." Andy hadn't meant for that to happen.

- Andy thought he used an "I" message when he spoke to Davis. What kind of message did he really send? What could Andy say now to restore the friendship?

____

____

____

____

____

____

____

B. Juanita is twelve years old and will be thirteen in less than six months. Her parents hire an older teen to baby-sit her one-year-old brother when they go out. Juanita feels that she is mature enough now to baby-sit her brother.

- What can Juanita say to persuade her parents to allow her to baby-sit?

____

____

____

____

____

____

____

Name ______________________

Vocabulary Reinforcement

Use Word Meanings

Decide whether each of the following sentences is correct. If it is correct, write *correct* on the line. If it is not correct, replace the italicized word or phrase with one from the box to make the sentence correct. Use each word or phrase only once. You will not use every one.

adolescence	**hormones**	**ovum**	**abstinence**
embryo	**nervous system**	**pituitary gland**	**muscular system**
heredity	**nucleus**	**skeletal system**	

1. The *skeletal system* directs and controls all movement in the body. ______________
2. The *fetus* develops in the uterus from two weeks until two months after fertilization. ______________
3. The *circulatory system* produces red blood cells. ______________
4. Growth hormone in girls is produced by the *ovaries.* ______________
5. The passing of traits from parents to children is *abstinence.* ______________
6. The organs of the *muscular system* move voluntarily and involuntarily. ______________
7. Glands produce *neurons* that control the functions of organs. ______________
8. The *chromosome* controls the division of material that duplicates itself in cell division. ______________
9. When you reach *maturity,* you will be fully developed. ______________
10. When you practice *abstinence* from alcohol and tobacco, you do not use them. ______________

CHAPTER 2

Name ______________________________

Quick Study

Personal and Consumer Health

Directions

- Use the vocabulary in the Word Bank to complete each **Summary**.
- Read the other directions to complete each **Lesson Details**.

Word Bank

acne	consumers	floss	reliable
advertising	decibels	ingredients	repetitive strain injuries
conjunctivitis	distraction	plaque	sties
			sunscreen

Lesson 1 pp. 42–47

Summary Caring for your skin, hair, and nails is important to good health. Clean skin helps prevent skin disorders, such as ______________. Using ______________ helps protect your skin from harmful UV rays in sunlight.

Lesson Details Use the photos on page 44 to explain what causes acne. Use these terms: *oil gland, dermis, pore, bacteria, pimple.* ______________________________

____

____

Lesson 2 pp. 48–53

Summary Wise ______________ do not believe everything they read or hear in ______________. They buy products based on their needs and the product's quality. They can get product details from the list of ______________ on the label.

Lesson Details Look at the label for Natural Deodorant Soap on page 52 in your textbook. Write an ad for the soap, using one of the tricks described on pages 48 and 49.

Lesson 3 pp. 56–59

Summary To properly care for your teeth and gums, you must remove ______________, the sticky substance that coats your teeth. Before you brush your teeth, ______________ to clean places on your teeth that a brush can't reach.

Name ______________________________ **Quick Study (continued)**

Lesson Details Complete the graphic organizer to show the steps that lead to tooth decay.

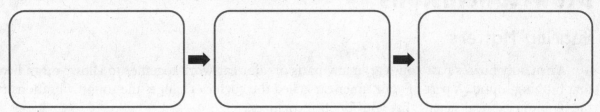

	➡		➡	

Lesson 4 pp. 60–64

Summary Vision and hearing are important senses that need to be protected. Common eye infections include ______________, which are caused by blocked hair follicles, and ______________, which is also called pinkeye. Sounds at or above 80 ______________ can harm your hearing.

Lesson Details Describe two ways to protect your eyes and two ways to protect your ears.

____

____

Lesson 5 pp. 66–69

Summary Do not let technology products become a ______________ from what is going on around you. Take breaks to avoid ____________________.

Lesson Details Complete the chart to show ways to stay safe while using a computer.

Head/Shoulders	Eyes	Arms/Hands	Legs/Feet

Lesson 6 pp. 70–74

Summary You need to use ______________ health information to make decisions about health products.

Lesson Details Suppose you need to decide which toothpaste to buy. What sources of information can you use to make your decision?

____

Name ___________________________

Focus Skill **Reading Skill**

Draw Conclusions

Hearing Matters

When a fly buzzes past your ear, many parts of your ear work together to allow you to hear that buzzing sound. A part of your inner ear called the cochlea changes the sound vibrations from the fly into electrical signals that your brain recognizes.

The cochlea is a small tube that is curled like a snail shell. Liquid fills the curled tube, and special hair cells line an inner membrane. Sound vibrations that reach the cochlea travel through the liquid. When the hair cells within the cochlea detect the liquid's movement, they change the vibrations into electrical signals. These electrical signals are sent through nerves to the brain, where they are recognized as sounds.

Different sounds cause the liquid in the cochlea to vibrate in different ways. The more forceful the vibrations, the more the hair cells move. Loud sounds cause strong vibrations to travel through your cochlea. If a sound is very loud, the vibrations may be strong enough to damage or break the hair cells. Damage to these hair cells can cause hearing loss. That is why it is important to protect your ears from loud sounds.

Using the graphic organizer, fill in the details and the conclusion.

What I Read:		What I Know:		Conclusion:
	+		=	

Name ________________________________

Problem Solving

Life Skill

Make Responsible Decisions

Steps for Making Responsible Decisions

1. Find out about the choices you could make.
2. Eliminate choices that are illegal or against your family's rules.
3. Ask yourself: What could happen with each choice? Does the choice show good character?
4. Make what seems to be the best choice.

Use the steps to tell how these students can make responsible decisions.

A. Henry's parents have explained that they don't want Henry to use health products without first talking to them or to a doctor. One day Henry's best friend, Miguel, shows him a skin product that he says not only cleans skin but prevents acne. Miguel says everyone is using the product. Both Henry and Miguel are developing acne, and Henry is interested in trying the product.

- What can Henry do to make a trustworthy and responsible decision?

____

____

____

____

B. Niomi just got braces to help straighten her teeth. Her dentist told her to brush her teeth after each meal to prevent cavities that might be caused by food trapped around her braces. Niomi brushes her teeth after meals at home, but she's embarrassed to brush her teeth at school. Niomi knows that most dentists recommend brushing teeth twice a day, so she decides that brushing twice a day at home is enough.

- Is Niomi's decision responsible? How could she do what her dentist asks?

____

____

____

____

____

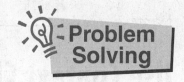

Name ___

Vocabulary Reinforcement

Use Context Clues

Read the following sentences. Use the context of the sentence to help you write a definition for the underlined word. Use your textbook to check your definition.

1. The injury to the skin was superficial, affecting only the epidermis.

___

2. Even though it was early morning, Sam wore sunscreen at the beach.

___

3. The advertising for the toothpaste made Maria interested in buying the product.

___

___

4. Plaque forms tartar when it hardens over time and can cause tooth decay.

___

5. When Mary said that she couldn't read the words on the board from the back of the classroom, her teacher concluded that Mary was nearsighted.

___

6. Listening to music at or above 80 decibels can cause hearing loss.

___

7. Aaron's doctor explained that playing his electronic game for hours had caused a repetitive strain injury.

___

8. Stacy knew that listening to her headphones was a distraction when she rode her bike.

___

CHAPTER 3

Name ______________________________

Quick Study

Preparing Healthful Foods

Directions

- Use the vocabulary in the Word Bank to complete each **Summary**.
- Use the section directions to complete the **Lesson Details**.

Word Bank

calories	bulimia	minerals	fats	staple
carbohydrates	vitamins	additives	anorexia	preservatives
fiber	proteins	balanced diet	vegetarian	
nutritional deficiency	convenience foods	cholesterol	MyPyramid	

Lesson 1 pp. 80–85

Summary The nutrients that give your body energy are ______________, ______________, and ______________. The amount of energy in food is measured in ______________. Calcium and iron are examples of ______________. ______________ are the nutrients that help chemical reactions take place in your body. A chewy material in some foods is ______________. ______________ is a substance found in fats.

Lesson Details Look at the information on page 83. On a separate sheet of paper, use the information to explain why it is important to eat a variety of foods each day.

Lesson 2 pp. 86–89

Summary A(n) ______________ contains a variety of foods. ______________ helps you plan healthful eating. A(n) ______________ does not eat foods that come from animals.

Lesson Details Use MyPyramid on page 87 to complete the table.

Food Group	Recommended Amount per Day
Milk	
Fruits	
Grains	

Name ______________________________

Lesson 3 pp. 90–95

Summary A(n) ______________ is a key food ingredient in a particular region or area.

Lesson Details Use the information on pages 90, 92, and 95 to complete the table.

Food	Meat & Beans Group	Oils	Vegetables Group
Chicken Soft Tacos	chicken		
Stir-Fried Tofu and Vegetables		stir-fry oil	
Beef Kebabs			tomatoes

Lesson 4 pp. 96–100

Summary An eating disorder that involves out-of-control dieting nearly to the point of starvation is called ______________. Eating a great deal of food and then vomiting right away is ______________, another eating disorder. The lack of a certain nutrient in the diet is a(n) ______________________.

Lesson Details Look at the information on page 99. What are the three main steps of the USDA's Dietary Guidelines?

____

Lesson 5 pp. 102–107

Summary Foods that are partly or completely prepared when you buy them are ______________. ______________ are substances added to foods to keep them fresh longer or to improve their color or flavor. Certain substances called ______________ help keep food from spoiling.

Lesson Details Use the information on page 104 to answer the question. If a food is labeled as low-fat and high-fiber, what is the maximum amount of fat in one serving?

____

Name ______________________________

Focus Skill **Reading Skill**

Compare and Contrast

Carbohydrates and Proteins

Your body needs many different nutrients to grow and stay healthy. Carbohydrates and proteins are both nutrients needed by your body. Along with fats, carbohydrates and proteins are the nutrients that your body uses for energy and growth.

Sugars and starches are carbohydrates. Foods such as whole grains, fruits, and vegetables are good sources of carbohydrates. Your body gets energy from carbohydrates. Some carbohydrates—simple carbohydrates—provide immediate energy for your body. Other carbohydrates—complex carbohydrates—provide energy for your body over a longer period of time.

Proteins are nutrients used by your body for building and repairing cells. Although proteins contain the same amount of energy per gram as carbohydrates, your body uses them in a different way. Proteins are used primarily for building the body. Proteins are found mainly in meats, poultry, fish, dried beans, eggs, and nuts.

Fill in the graphic organizer by telling how carbohydrates and proteins are alike and how they are different.

Compare and Contrast

Alike	Different

Name ______________________

Problem Solving

Life Skill

Make Responsible Decisions

Steps for Making Responsible Decisions

1. Find out about the choices you could make.
2. Eliminate choices that are against your family rules.
3. Ask yourself: What is the possible result of each choice? Does the choice show good character?
4. Make what seems to be the best choice.

Use the steps to help these students make responsible decisions.

A. Keyona's family has gone to a restaurant for a healthful dinner. There are many choices of foods on the menu. They include cheeseburgers with fries, baked chicken with baked potato, and lasagna with meat sauce. After Keyona studies the menu, she decides to order a cheeseburger and french fries.

- Was Keyona's decision to order a cheeseburger and french fries healthful and responsible? Why or why not? If Keyona did not make a healthful and responsible choice, tell what a better choice would have been.

____

____

____

____

____

B. After school Lee has football practice. Lee wants to find a snack that will give him quick energy for exercising. He stops at the corner market on the way to football practice to buy a snack. Lee's family has a rule that all snacks must be healthful.

- Explain how Lee can choose a healthful snack that will give him quick energy. Make sure to explain how Lee's choice can help him follow his family's rules.

____

____

____

____

____

Name ______________________________

Vocabulary Reinforcement

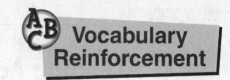

Use Word Meanings

Match the definitions with the words in the box. Write the letter of the correct word on the line by the definition.

a. fiber	**d. vitamin**	**g. calories**	**j. MyPyramid**
b. fats	**e. protein**	**h. carbohydrates**	**k. staple**
c. mineral	**f. cholesterol**	**i. vegetarian**	**l. additive**

____ **1.** Key food ingredient of a region or an area

____ **2.** Nutrients that yield the most calories per gram

____ **3.** Substance added to foods to keep them fresh or to improve color or flavor

____ **4.** Nutrient used primarily to build and repair cells

____ **5.** Nutrient that does not provide energy but helps the body grow and work

____ **6.** A food guide pyramid that can help you develop a personal plan for healthful eating and physical activity

____ **7.** Substance found in fats; high levels are associated with heart disease

____ **8.** Chewy or gritty substance in food; this material is not a nutrient

____ **9.** Units in which the amount of energy in food is measured

____ **10.** Nutrients used for energy—sugars and starches

____ **11.** Person who does not eat foods that come from animals

____ **12.** Nutrient that helps chemical reactions take place in the body

CHAPTER 4

Name ______________________________

Quick Study

Keeping Active

Directions

- Use lesson vocabulary in the Word Bank to complete each **Summary**. You will not use all of the terms.
- Use the directions provided to complete each **Lesson Details**.

Word Bank

Activity Pyramid	cardiovascular fitness	hyperthermia	warm-up	workout
aerobic exercise	cool-down	hypothermia	muscular strength	
anaerobic exercise	flexibility	muscular endurance	target heart rate	

Lesson 1 pp. 120–125

Summary Different types of exercise produce different results. Exercises such as lifting weights and doing push-ups will help you gain ______________________. If you use your muscles a lot, you will gain ______________________. Stretching can help you gain ______________________, the ability to move your body from one position to another. Most important, exercises such as swimming and fast walking will help you gain ______________________, an important part of physical fitness.

Lesson Details Use the calorie chart on page 123 to help you complete the chart.

Calories Used by a 99-Pound Person

Activity/Time	Calories Used
Basketball ($\frac{1}{2}$ hour) and Tennis ($\frac{1}{2}$ hour)	
Dancing (2 hours)	
Climbing stairs ($\frac{1}{2}$ hour) and Skating ($\frac{1}{2}$ hour)	

Name ______________________________ **Quick Study (continued)**

Lesson 2 pp. 128–134

Summary Each ______________ should begin with a ______________ exercise and end with a ______________ exercise. ______________ helps to build cardiovascular fitness. You need to reach your ______________ to gain a benefit. ______________ mainly helps build muscle strength.

Lesson Details Reread page 134. Tell why it is important to get enough sleep.

____

____

Lesson 3 pp. 136–140

Summary You should avoid exercising outside when it is very cold or very hot. When it is very hot, you risk getting heat stroke, the most serious form of ______________. When it is very cold, you might get an illness called ______________. Signs of this illness include shivering, slurred speech, confusion, and drowsiness.

Lesson Details Use the information on pages 136–137 to help you complete the graphic organizer.

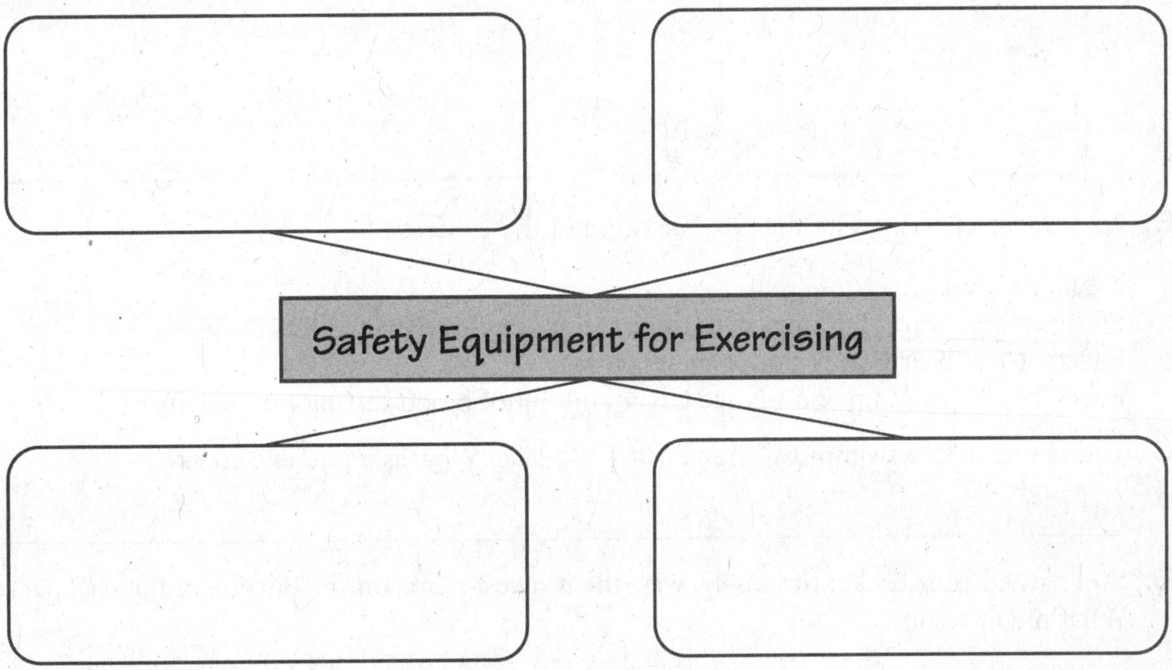

Name ______________________________

Focus Skill **Reading Skill**

Identify Cause and Effect

A. Supply a possible effect or effects for each of the following causes.

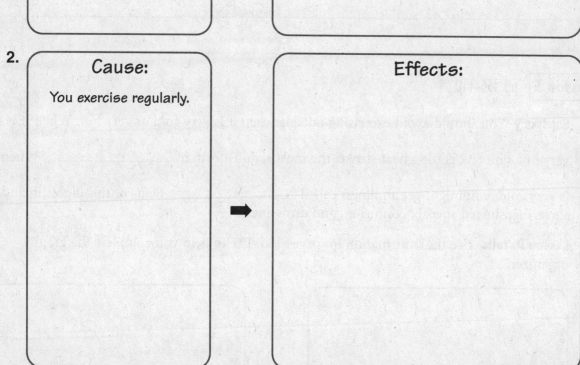

1.

Cause:		Effects:
You don't exercise.	➡	

2.

Cause:		Effects:
You exercise regularly.	➡	

B. Look at the effects. Write the possible cause of these effects.

Possible Cause: ______________________________
Effect: strong heart and lungs over time
Effect: at-rest heartbeat is slower than before
Effect: heart speeds up and pumps larger amount of blood during this activity

C. You ignore a "No swimming" sign posted at a lake. What is a possible effect?

____

D. You packed your backpack loosely, with the heaviest items on the outside of the backpack. What might result?

____

Name ______________________________

Problem Solving

Life Skill

Set Goals

Steps for Setting Goals

1. Choose a goal.
2. List and plan steps to meet the goal. Determine how long it will take.
3. Check your progress as you work toward the goal.
4. Reflect on and evaluate your progress.

Use the steps to help these students set goals for fitness.

A. Jeremy wants to lose five pounds. Although he exercises regularly, he never seems to be able to lose weight.

- Explain how Jeremy can use goal setting to help him lose the five pounds.

____

____

____

____

____

____

____

B. Elizabeth has an important tennis match in one month. She wants to win the match, but she is not in the best physical condition. She is afraid she will become very tired if the match lasts too long.

- Describe how Elizabeth can use goal setting to increase her chances of winning the match.

____

____

____

____

____

____

Name ______________________________

ABC **Vocabulary Reinforcement**

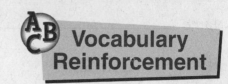

Find the Meaning

A. Match the terms in Column B with the definitions in Column A. Write the letters in the spaces provided. Use each term only once.

	Column A	**Column B**
1. ____	Illness that can occur in cold weather	**a.** muscular strength
2. ____	What you gain when you use your muscles to push, pull, or lift heavy objects	**b.** muscular endurance
3. ____	The heart rate at which your heart and lungs become stronger	**c.** cardiovascular fitness
4. ____	Builds a healthy heart and lungs	**d.** target heart rate
5. ____	What you gain when you use your muscles for long periods	**e.** aerobic exercise
6. ____	Name given to several heat-related illnesses	**f.** anaerobic exercise
7. ____	Ability to move your body from position to position	**g.** warm-up
8. ____	The first part of a workout	**h.** hyperthermia
9. ____	Means that your heart, lungs, and circulatory system work well	**i.** hypothermia
10. ____	Short, intense activities such as lifting weights	**j.** flexibility

B. Write a paragraph using each of these words: *workout, warm-up, cool-down.*

____

____

____

____

____

____

CHAPTER 5 Name ______________________________

Quick Study

Staying Safe Every Day

Directions

- Use the chapter vocabulary in the Word Bank to complete each **Summary**.
- Read the section directions to complete each **Lesson Details**.

Word Bank

electric shock, fire hazard, flammable, gang, poison, reach and throw, survival floating, terrorism, weapon

Lesson 1 pp. 146–151

Summary You can be safe at home. To prevent ______________, follow safety rules when using electricity. Properly store ______________ materials to prevent fires. Know safety rules to avoid a ______________, a dangerous situation that might result in a fire.

Lesson Details Copy the graphic organizer onto another sheet of paper. Use pages 150–151 to complete the graphic organizer by listing three safety rules in each box.

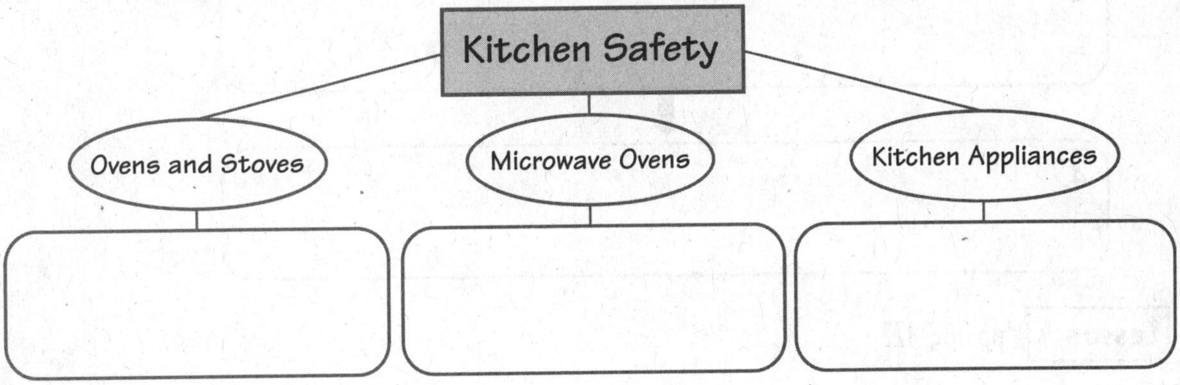

Lesson 2 pp. 152–158

Summary Personal safety depends on taking precautions. Avoid (1) dangerous situations; (2) dangerous objects, such as a ______________, that could injure or kill a person; and (3) harmful materials, such as ______________.

Lesson Details Suppose that you are going to baby-sit your neighbors' first-grade son for an evening. What questions will you ask before the parents leave? What will you do to make sure the first-grader stays safe while the parents are gone?

____

____

Lesson 3 pp. 160–165

Summary In a water emergency, remember to use ____________________, a lifesaving technique that can help people at risk of drowning. If you are caught in deep, warm water, use ____________________ to increase your chances of survival.

Lesson Details Use the graphic organizer below to show the steps in survival floating and the details about how to do each step.

1.

↓

2.

↓

3.

↓

4.

Lesson 4 pp. 168–172

Summary People can avoid conflicts and survive violence in many ways, including by avoiding ________________ membership. Also important is following emergency guidelines during public violence, such as acts of ________________.

Lesson Details Suppose that a friend tells you that he does not feel safe in his neighborhood, has been pressured to join a gang, and feels confused about how he should protect himself. Use the space below to explain what you would tell your friend.

____

____

____

Name ______________________________

Focus Skill **Reading Skill**

Identify Main Idea and Details

The Shocking Details of Electricity

Imagine what your home would be like without electricity—no stove, refrigerator, television, lights, or fans. Electricity is a very useful part of your life, but with its benefits also come some dangers. Knowing how to use electricity safely is important.

To stay safe with electricity, look for warning signs that can alert you to dangerous electrical situations. In your home, look for damage to the plastic or rubber coating on electrical cords. A damaged electrical cord could cause a fire or an electric shock. Look for water before using an electrical appliance. If water is near, move the appliance to a dry area before using it. Finally, make sure that electrical outlets are not overloaded and that empty outlets have protective covers to prevent accidental injuries.

One of the most dangerous outdoor electrical hazards is a downed electrical wire. Sometimes winds or storms cause a power line to snap and fall to the ground. If you see a downed power line, stay far away from it. Touching the power line or an object in contact with it could cause severe injuries or death. Also, look out for trees with branches that are near power lines. When a tree grows near a power line, it can damage the line and cause electric shock hazards, power outages, and fire hazards. Do not climb or play near trees that have branches near power lines.

If you notice any of these hazards in or around your home, tell a responsible adult as soon as possible. You may help prevent a serious electrical accident.

Using the graphic organizer, fill in the main idea and details about electrical safety inside and outside the home.

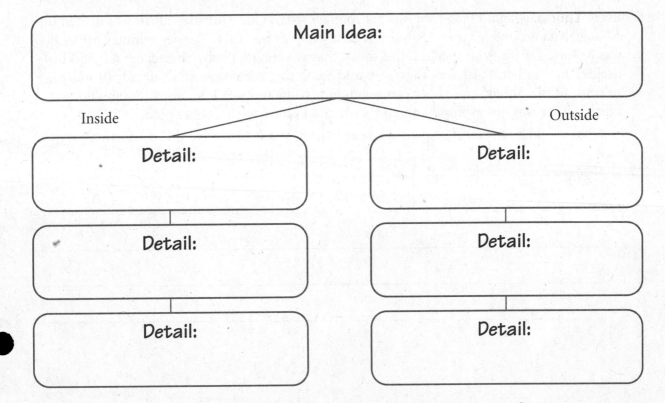

Main Idea:

Inside	Outside
Detail:	Detail:
Detail:	Detail:
Detail:	Detail:

Name ______________________

Problem Solving

Life Skill

Resolve Conflicts

Steps for Resolving Conflicts

1. Use "I" messages to tell how you feel.
2. Listen to each other. Consider the other person's point of view.
3. Negotiate.
4. Compromise on a solution.

Use the steps to help these students resolve their conflicts.

A. Eddie and Samantha are the two best soccer players on their team. The day the team voted for captain, Samantha was responsible for the after-practice snack and brought fresh fruit for the team. When she was named captain, Eddie was furious. He thought the vote was unfair and that Samantha had bribed the team for votes. Samantha was angered by the accusation, saying she hadn't made the schedule showing she should bring snacks that day.

- Explain how Eddie and Samantha might resolve their conflict.

____

____

____

____

____

B. Every Thursday night Elijah baby-sits his younger sister. One Thursday Elijah was invited to a baseball game, and his friend Sarah agreed to baby-sit his sister. Twenty minutes before he was to leave for the game, Sarah called to say that she couldn't baby-sit because a friend had decided to visit her. Elijah was angry. He told Sarah that because she had already promised to baby-sit, she should cancel her plans with her friend and watch his sister. Sarah said that Elijah's sister was his responsibility, so she shouldn't have to cancel her plans.

- What would be the most respectful and trustworthy way to resolve this conflict?

____

____

____

____

____

Name ______________________

Vocabulary Reinforcement

Use Word Meanings

Choose the BEST word from the box to complete each sentence.

electric shock	flammable	fire hazard	poison	
weapon	reach and throw	survival floating	gang	terrorism

1. As an emergency room doctor, Manuel's mother sees people who have swallowed ______________________ and need immediate medical care.

2. Alan was relieved when his older brother decided not to become a member of a neighborhood ______________________.

3. Li An stored the rubbing alcohol in a cool pantry away from a heat source because it is a ______________________ material.

4. Public violence that involves people who use violence for social or political reasons is ______________________.

5. Alicia told her younger brother that he should not light candles in his room because they create a ______________________.

6. In Erika's swimming class, she learned ______________________ as a way to conserve energy if caught in deep, warm water.

7. In Noah's school district, any elementary, middle, or high school student who brings a ______________________ to school is suspended or expelled.

8. An electrician replaced the damaged cord on Mrs. Alsted's vacuum cleaner to prevent anyone from getting an ______________________.

9. When Maria fell into the water, Josh used ______________________ to help her out of the water and keep her from drowning.

CHAPTER 6

Name ______________________________

Quick Study

Emergencies and First Aid

Directions

- Use lesson vocabulary in the Word Bank to complete each **Summary**.
- Read the directions provided to complete each **Lesson Details**.

Word Bank

abdominal thrusts	fracture	hypothermia	shock
disaster	frostbite	rescue breathing	sprain
first aid	hyperthermia	seizure	supply kit

Lesson 1 pp. 178–183

Summary A ______________, such as a hurricane, calls for emergency action. You can prepare for such an emergency by making family plans, organizing an emergency ______________ and a first-aid kit, and having emergency telephone information on hand.

Lesson Details Use pages 180–183 to complete the graphic organizer.

Reducing the Risks of Disasters

Fire	Blizzard	Hurricane
Tornado	Earthquake	Severe Thunderstorm

Lesson 2 pp. 186–192

Summary A rescuer can use ______________ to help an injured person before medical help arrives. Common injuries for which treatment may be needed include a ______________, a ______________, a sports injury, a burn, a ______________, ______________, ______________, and ______________.

Lesson Details Look at pages 187–188. Describe and explain the importance of each step of the RICE treatment.

Rest ____

Ice ____

____

Compress ____

____

Elevate ____

____

____

Lesson 3 pp. 194–200

Summary Life-threatening emergencies require immediate attention. A rescuer may need to administer ____________ for a person who is choking. ____________ can save a person whose breathing has stopped. A rescuer may need to keep a person suffering from ____________ lying down and comfortable.

Lesson Details Use the information on pages 194–200 to fill in the chart.

Emergency	Signs	First-Aid Treatment
	Inability to breathe, cough, or talk; clutching the throat with both hands	Perform one or more abdominal thrusts.
Stopped Breathing		Perform rescue breathing.
Severe Bleeding	Blood spurting, flowing, or oozing out of a wound	
Shock		Call 911. Keep the person lying down with feet and legs elevated.
Poisoning	Burns or stains around mouth, nausea, drowsiness	

Name ______________________________

Focus Skill **Reading Skill**

Summarize

Responding to an Emergency

When Teri and her family moved into their new home, one of the first things they did was to make a plan to escape their house in case of fire. They knew the plan might come in handy to save their lives, but they didn't realize it would be so soon.

The night after the family's discussion, a hot-water heater in a downstairs closet caught fire. The fire was contained in the closet for a short while but suddenly erupted into flames that engulfed the hallway leading to the parents' bedroom. Smoke quickly filled the downstairs area, setting off the alarms throughout the house.

Luckily, everyone was awakened by the alarms. Teri and her sister rushed from their upstairs bedrooms, meeting their brother in the hallway. Smoke had begun to drift into the upstairs area, and they were concerned about going downstairs, where the smoke was dense and where the fire was. Instead, they decided to leave the house through a window at the end of the hallway. That would give them easy access to a porch roof and then the ground below.

Reaching the ground, they ran toward the sidewalk, where the family had decided to meet in case of evacuation. The children were concerned for their parents but followed the escape plan as they had all discussed it. Suddenly, the children heard their father's voice as he and their mother approached them from the side yard. Their parents had narrowly escaped the flames by slipping out of a side window.

Tearfully, they huddled together briefly, before Teri's mother ran to a neighbor's home to call for emergency help. They had all wanted to practice their plan, but now they had used it for a real escape. They were thankful that their plan had worked and all were safe.

Summarize the correct safety procedures the family used.

____

____

____

____

____

____

____

Name ____________________

Problem Solving

Life Skill

Communicate

Steps for Effective Communication

1. Understand your audience.
2. Give a clear message. Express ideas in a clear, organized way.
3. Listen carefully, and answer any questions.
4. Follow directions.

Use the steps to help these students communicate in an effective way.

A. Sean is riding with his mother when they see a serious accident involving several cars. Sean's mother tells Sean to call 911 as she rushes to assist the cars' occupants.

- Explain what information Sean should give the 911 operator when he makes the call.

____

____

____

____

____

____

B. Trish is baby-sitting a neighbor's child who has been ill. The child's mother tells Trish where she will be and how to reach her if there are any problems. She also points out a list of other emergency contacts, including the doctor who is caring for the child.

- An hour after the mother leaves, the child complains of a headache and begins vomiting. Trish calls the mother, who says she will be right home, but she asks that Trish call the doctor to determine how to help the child. Explain how Trish could act responsibly to get appropriate help for the child.

____

____

____

____

____

____

____

Name ________________________________

Vocabulary Reinforcement

Use Word Meanings

A. In each of the following sentences, the underlined term makes the sentence incorrect. Look in the box to find the term that makes the sentence correct. Write the correct term on the line. Use each term only once.

abdominal thrusts	**first aid**	**hyperthermia**	**shock**
disaster	**frostbite**	**hypothermia**	**sprain**

1. A condition in which the body temperature becomes too low is shock. ____________
2. For a choking person who is unable to breathe, cough, or speak, rescue breathing would be the appropriate treatment. ____________
3. Immediate care given to someone who is injured or ill is called hospitalization. ____________
4. A severe thunderstorm that results in a great amount of damage to an area is a blizzard. ____________
5. A condition in which body tissue freezes is referred to as hypothermia. ____________
6. Another name for heatstroke is sunburn. ____________
7. Elevating the feet is a step to take when a person is in denial. ____________
8. An injury caused by the twisting of a joint is called a fracture. ____________

B. Write a sentence about each of the terms below.

1. seizure

____

2. fracture

____

3. rescue breathing

____

CHAPTER 7

Name ______________________________

Quick Study

Controlling Disease

Directions

- Use the vocabulary and other terms in the Word Bank to complete each **Summary**.
- Use the section directions to complete the **Lesson Details**.

Word Bank

cardiovascular disease	sexually transmitted diseases (STDs)	insulin	immune system	antibodies
vaccine	toxins	abstinence	pathogen	immunization
antibiotic	resistance	stress	immunity	boosters
communicable disease	noncommunicable diseases	health risk factor	carcinogens	infection

Lesson 1 pp. 206–211

Summary Any condition that increases your chances of becoming ill is a(n) ______________________. A(n) ______________________ is an organism or a virus that can make you sick.

Lesson Details Describe each type of health risk factor.

1. Hereditary risk factors: ______________________

2. Environmental risk factors: ______________________

____

3. Behavioral risk factors: ______________________

____

Lesson 2 pp. 214–221

Summary Any disease that can spread from person to person is a(n) ______________________. Diseases spread by sexual contact are called ______________________. The only way for a young person to avoid STDs is to practice ______________________. Pathogens multiplying in your body can cause ______________________. Pathogens called bacteria produce ______________________, or wastes, that can make you ill.

Name ________________________________

Quick Study (continued)

Lesson Details Use the information on page 215 to list an example of a disease in the table.

Pathogen	Viruses	Bacteria	Fungi	Protozoa
Disease				

Lesson 3 pp. 222–227

Summary Your body has ____________, or a natural ability to fight pathogens. The body system that recognizes and destroys pathogens is the ____________. It produces white blood cells, which make ____________ to fight disease. Your body has ____________ to any pathogens it has already fought. A(n) ____________ is a dose of a(n) ____________. ____________ are later doses. A(n) ____________ is a medicine that kills pathogens.

Lesson Details On a separate sheet of paper, list three of the body's defenses. Tell how each protects the body.

Lesson 4 pp. 228–234

Summary ________________________ can't be spread from person to person. One type of these, ________________________, affects the heart. Substances that cause cancer are called ____________. In the disease diabetes, ____________ is not made or is not used properly.

Lesson Details Write a sentence that tells the relationship between cancer and carcinogens.

____

Lesson 5 pp. 236–240

Summary ____________ lowers a person's natural resistance to disease.

Lesson Details List three ways to handle stress healthfully.

1. ____________________ 2. ____________________

3. ____

Name ______________________

Focus Skill **Reading Skill**

Compare and Contrast

Risk Factors

A health risk factor is any factor that increases the risk of disease. There are several types, or categories, of risk factors.

Hereditary risk factors are inherited traits that increase your chances of becoming ill. You don't have any control over hereditary risk factors. Some forms of heart disease are hereditary. Sickle cell anemia is also a disease that is hereditary.

Behavioral health risks are harmful behaviors that increase your chances of becoming ill. You have control over behavioral risk factors. Using tobacco is an example of a behavioral risk factor. This behavior increases your chances of getting cancer and other diseases.

Fill in the graphic organizer by telling how hereditary risk factors and behavioral risk factors are alike and how they are different. Provide an example of each.

Compare and Contrast

Alike	Different

Name ______________________________

Problem Solving

Life Skill

Manage Stress

Steps for Managing Stress

1. Know what stress feels like.
2. Try to determine the cause of your stress.
3. Talk to someone about the way you're feeling.
4. Do something to help relieve your stress.

Use the steps to help these students manage stress.

A. Tara has been worried about her math test all week. Although she has studied, she does not feel that she will do well. All week she has been overeating when she thinks about the test.

- Use the steps for managing stress to help Tara respond to her stress in a positive way.

____

____

____

____

____

____

B. Juan has been invited to hang out with a group of older teens in his neighborhood. He knows that all of the teens in the group smoke. He is feeling stress because he does not want to start smoking just to fit in with the group.

- Use the steps for managing stress to help Juan respond to his stress in a positive way.

____

____

____

____

____

____

Name ___________________________

Vocabulary Reinforcement

Choose the Correct Term

Read each sentence, and underline the term that makes it true.

1. Colds and flu are both [communicable diseases/noncommunicable diseases].
2. Bacteria can produce wastes called [insulin/toxins] that can make you ill.
3. Your immune system makes [abstinence/antibodies], which fight disease.
4. If you have diabetes, your body can't use or make [insulin/carcinogens] properly.
5. Syphilis and gonorrhea are [sexually transmitted diseases/noncommunicable diseases].
6. Air pollution is a(n) [behavioral risk factor/environmental risk factor].
7. Fungi and protozoa are both types of [carcinogens/pathogens].
8. Additional doses of vaccines, called [antibiotics/boosters], can be given at a later time to help you stay immune to some diseases.
9. A [symptom/resistance] is a sign or feeling of having a disease.
10. The only sure way for a young person to protect himself or herself from sexually transmitted diseases is to practice [resistance/abstinence].
11. Your body's ability to defend itself against pathogens that you have already been exposed to is called [immunity/disease].
12. An [immune system/immunization] is a dose of a vaccine.
13. Heart disease is a [cardiovascular disease/communicable disease].

CHAPTER 8

Name ______________________________

Quick Study

Drugs and Health

Directions

- Use lesson vocabulary in the Word Bank to complete each **Summary**.
- Read the section directions to complete each **Lesson Details**.

Word Bank

depressants	drug abuse	inhalants	prescription medicines
stimulants	dependence	marijuana	over-the-counter medicines
steroids	tolerance	refuse	drug

Lesson 1 pp. 246–251

Summary Any substance that changes the way your mind or body works is called a

________________. Medicines that doctors order are ________________.

Medicines available on store shelves are ________________.

Lesson Details Look at page 249. Explain the differences and similarities between prescription medicines and over-the-counter medicines.

____

____

____

Lesson 2 pp. 252–256

Summary ________________ is the improper use of medicine or the use of an illegal drug.

When users feel they need drugs to feel normal, they have developed ________________.
When users need more of a drug than they first did to get the same effect, they have

developed ________________.

Lesson Details Use the list of drug effects on pages 252–253 to complete the chart.

Effect	Symptoms
Health Effects	
Withdrawal	
Overdose	

Lesson 3 pp. 258–261

Summary ______________ are drugs that speed up brain activity and increase heart rate and blood pressure. Drugs that slow down brain activity and decrease heart rate are ______________. ______________ are hormone drugs, prescribed by doctors.

Lesson Details Use pages 258–259 to complete the graphic organizer.

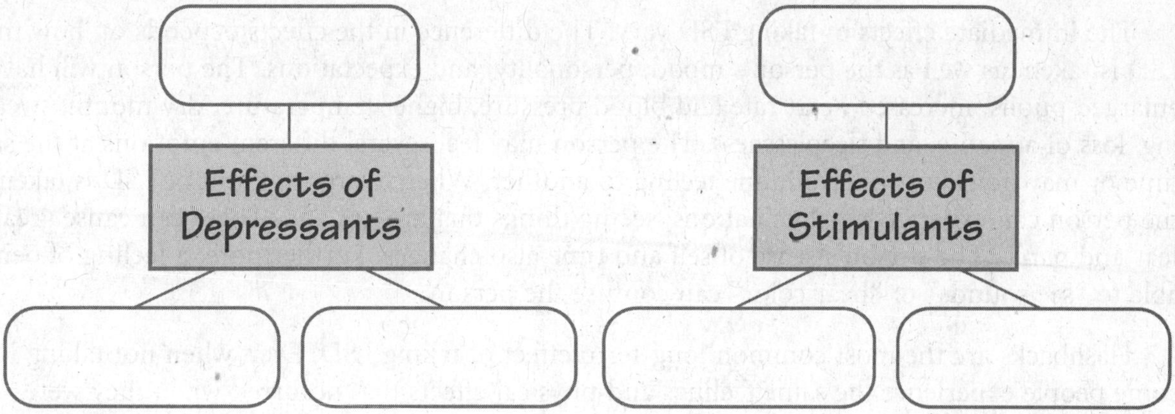

Lesson 4 pp. 262–267

Summary ______________ is the most common illegal drug in the United States. ______________ are also commonly abused.

Lesson Details Use the information on pages 263 and 266 to complete the chart.

Body Part	Effects of Marijuana	Effects of Inhalants
Brain		
Heart		
Muscles		

Lesson 5 pp. 270–274

Summary It is your right and responsibility to ______________ to take drugs. By knowing about drugs and by learning strategies for avoiding them, you can say no to drugs.

Lesson Details Look at "Where to Get Help in Refusing Drugs" on page 273. Describe two strategies you could use to help you refuse drugs.

____

____

Name ____________________

Focus Skill **Reading Skill**

Summarize

LSD

LSD is the most common hallucinogen and a powerful mood-altering drug.

LSD comes from an acid found in a type of fungus. The acid is manufactured into colored tablets, blotter paper, clear liquid, and squares of gelatin. Users of LSD either swallow a tablet, lick it off blotter paper, or put the liquid or gelatin squares in their eyes.

The immediate effects of taking LSD vary. The difference in the effects depends on how much LSD is taken, as well as the person's mood, personality, and expectations. The person will have enlarged pupils, increased heart rate and blood pressure, higher temperature, dry mouth, sweating, loss of appetite, and sleeplessness. The person may feel several different emotions at the same time or may quickly swing from one feeling to another. When a large amount of LSD is taken, the person can experience hallucinations, seeing things that are not real. These can cause great fear and panic. The person's sense of self and time also changes. Furthermore, a feeling of being able to "see sounds" or "hear color" can confuse the person.

Flashbacks are the most common long-term effect of taking LSD. Even when not taking it, some people experience the same feelings and physical effects that occurred when they were taking LSD. Such flashbacks can occur within days of taking LSD or more than a year later. A flashback generally happens without warning.

Although LSD is not an addictive drug, the side effects of taking it are serious. They include acting in ways the person normally would not, experiencing irrational emotions, experiencing bodily damage, and possibly suffering flashbacks.

Complete the graphic organizer to summarize the reading.

Main Idea:		Details:		Summary:
	+		=	

Name ____________________

Problem Solving

Life Skill

Refuse

Steps for Refusing to Use Drugs

1. Say *no* firmly. State your reasons for saying *no*.
2. Avoid possible problem situations.
3. Stay with people who also refuse to take part in harmful activities.
4. Ignore the person.

Use the steps to describe how these students can refuse to use drugs.

A. Tessa and Lisa decide to go to a community dance at the park. While they are there, two older boys invite them to join them. The boys then begin to smoke marijuana and offer some to the girls. How can the girls say no to smoking marijuana?

- Describe how Tessa and Lisa can say *no* to smoking marijuana by using refusal skills.

____

____

____

____

____

____

B. Max recently moved to a new neighborhood. When he went over to Marcus's house, Marcus showed him a bottle of his father's prescription pain pills, oxycodone. Marcus told Max that he will feel great if he tries one of the pills. How can Max say no to taking oxycodone?

- Describe how Max can use refusal skills to say *no* to Marcus.

____

____

____

____

____

____

Name ______________________________

Vocabulary Reinforcement

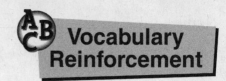

Match the Meanings

A. Match a definition in Column A with a word in Column B. Write the letter of the correct word on the line. Use each word only once.

Column A	Column B
1. ____ hormone drugs that are prescribed by doctors	**a.** inhalants
2. ____ powerful drugs, such as morphine, that relieve pain	**b.** hallucinogens
3. ____ drugs that slow down the activity of the brain	**c.** steroids
4. ____ the amount of a drug a patient should take	**d.** narcotics
5. ____ strong drugs that greatly increase brain activity	**e.** amphetamines
6. ____ illegal drugs that distort senses and affect the brain	**f.** depressants
7. ____ products whose poisonous fumes are breathed in	**g.** stimulants
8. ____ drugs that speed up the way the brain works, increase heart rate, and increase blood pressure	**h.** dosage

B. Choose two of the vocabulary words from Column B. Write a sentence comparing the drugs they name.

____

____

____

____

____

CHAPTER 9 Name ______________________________ Quick Study

Tobacco and Alcohol

Directions

- Use the vocabulary in the Word Bank to complete each **Summary**.
- Use the section directions to complete each **Lesson Details**.

Word Bank

alcohol-abuse counselors	blood alcohol level	intoxicated	recovery programs	tars
alcoholic	carbon monoxide	nicotine	self-respect	tobacco
alcoholism	environmental tobacco smoke (ETS)	negative peer pressure	smokeless tobacco	

Lesson 1 pp. 280–283

Summary The leaves from the ____________________ plant are used for smoking and chewing. The poison ____________________ is found in tobacco, and the poisonous gas ____________________ is found in tobacco smoke. Tobacco smoke also contains ____________________, which get trapped in smokers' lungs.

Lesson Details Use page 282 to complete this graphic organizer.

Harmful Effects of Smoking

- skin
- brain
- lungs
- throat
- mouth
- heart

Lesson 2 pp. 284–286

Summary Tobacco smoke harms nonsmokers who inhale ______________________________. Using ______________________________ is as dangerous as smoking cigarettes.

Name ______________________________

Lesson Details List three dangers of using smokeless tobacco. ____________________

____

____

____

Lesson 3 pp. 288–293

Summary The amount of alcohol in a person's body is the ____________________.

As the level of alcohol rises in a person's body, the person becomes ____________________.

____________________ develops when a person has an addiction to alcohol. A person with an addiction to alcohol is called a(n) ____________________.

Lesson Details Use page 290 to complete the graphic organizer.

Cause: Drinking too much alcohol → **Effect:**

Lesson 4 pp. 294–299

Summary Other young people may try to persuade you to use alcohol or tobacco. This is called ____________________. But when you value yourself as a person, you have ____________________ and have the strength to say *no* to tobacco and alcohol use.

Lesson Details Use another sheet of paper to answer this question. Why do advertisers spend large amounts of money on ads aimed at young people? Why is their advertising inaccurate?

Lesson 5 pp. 302–306

Summary ____________________ are people who work with alcoholics and their families to help them quit drinking. ____________________, found in hospitals and other places in the community, also help people stop using alcohol.

Lesson Details List three warning signs of problem drinkers.

____

____

Name ______________________________

Focus Skill **Reading Skill**

Identify Cause and Effect

Risks of Using Tobacco

Did you know that tobacco smoke contains at least 4,000 different ingredients? Forty-three of these ingredients are known carcinogens. Carcinogens are chemicals known to cause cancer. That means that every time someone smokes a cigarette, he or she is putting forty-three known cancer-causing chemicals into his or her mouth, throat, lungs, and bloodstream. By smoking, people automatically increase the risk of mouth, throat, larynx, esophageal, and lung cancers.

Another disease smokers may develop is emphysema. In fact, one-half—50 percent—of all smokers who continue to smoke after they get emphysema or certain types of cancer die because of these tobacco-related diseases.

Children are especially susceptible to the dangers of tobacco. When a pregnant woman uses tobacco, her unborn child is affected by the carcinogens that enter her bloodstream. Babies born to mothers who use tobacco are likely to be born prematurely or have a low birth weight. Both of those conditions are dangerous to newborn babies. Children who grow up in households where tobacco is used are exposed to environmental tobacco smoke. Environmental tobacco smoke has many negative effects on children, including increased incidences of asthma and other illnesses.

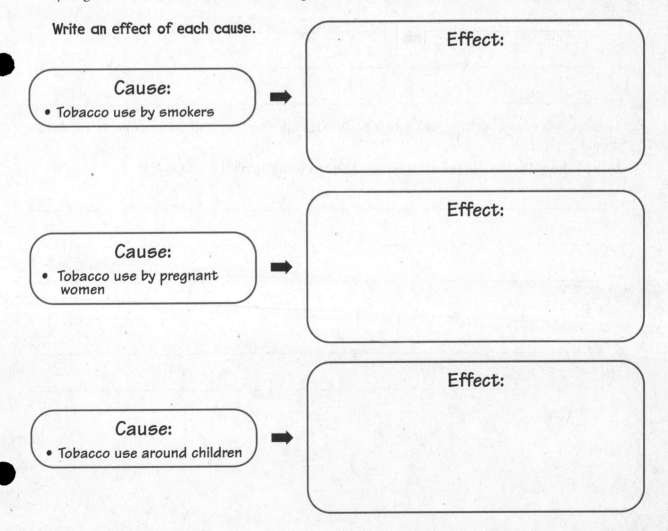

Write an effect of each cause.

Cause:
- Tobacco use by smokers

➡ **Effect:**

Cause:
- Tobacco use by pregnant women

➡ **Effect:**

Cause:
- Tobacco use around children

➡ **Effect:**

Name ______________________________

Problem Solving

Life Skill

Refuse

Steps for Refusing Alcohol and Tobacco

1. Say *no*.
2. Suggest something else to do.
3. Reverse the peer pressure.
4. Leave the situation.

Use the steps to help these students refuse alcohol and tobacco use.

A. James is at his friend Dylan's house while Dylan's parents are at work. While the boys are hanging out, Dylan opens a package of his mother's cigarettes and offers one to James. What should James do?

- Write how James can use refusal skills to say *no* to using tobacco.

____

____

____

____

____

____

B. Tia is at Sara's house getting ready for a party. Sara opens a beer and offers some to Tia. What should Tia do?

- Write how Tia can use refusal skills to say *no* to using alcohol.

____

____

____

____

____

____

Name ______________________________

Vocabulary Reinforcement

Crossword Puzzle

A. Use the clues to complete the crossword puzzle.

Across

1. a plant with large leaves used for smoking or chewing
2. a poisonous gas found in tobacco smoke
7. tobacco that is chewed or sucked rather than smoked
8. abbreviation for the amount of alcohol in a person's blood
9. another word for *drunk*

Down

1. substance that forms a thick layer in the lungs when tobacco is smoked
3. the disease that affects people who cannot control their use of alcohol
4. an addictive poison in tobacco
5. a person who is dependent on alcohol
6. abbreviation for smoke that is inhaled by nonsmokers

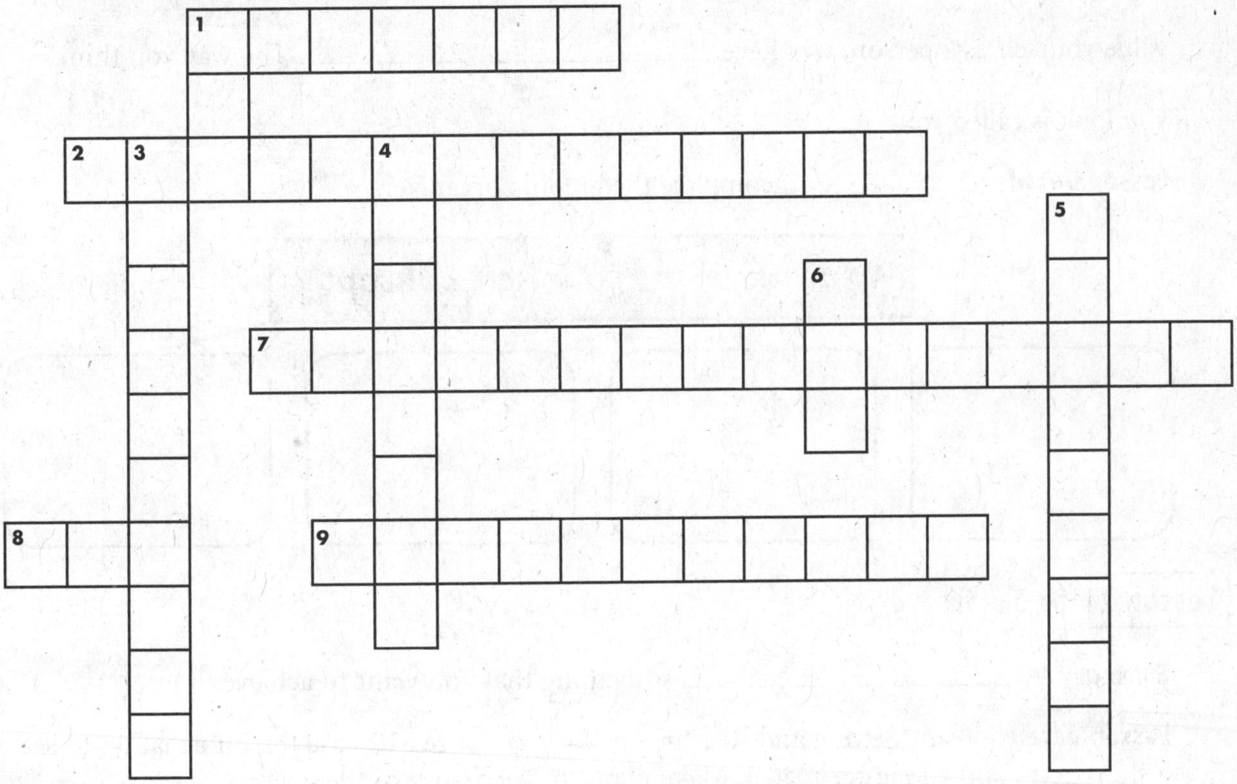

B. Choose two of the vocabulary words from Part A. Use the two words in a single sentence.

____

____

____

____

CHAPTER 10

Name ______________________________

Quick Study

Setting Goals

Directions

- Use lesson vocabulary in the Word Bank to complete each **Summary**.
- Read the other directions to complete each **Lesson Details**.

Word Bank

aggression	conflict resolution	peer pressure	self-concept	stereotype
body image	goal	prejudice	self-control	stress
conflict	peers	relaxation	self-respect	

Lesson 1 pp. 312–315

Summary The way you see yourself is your ______________________. When you value yourself as a person, you have ______________________. The way you think you look is called your ______________________.

Lesson Details Use page 312 to complete the graphic organizer.

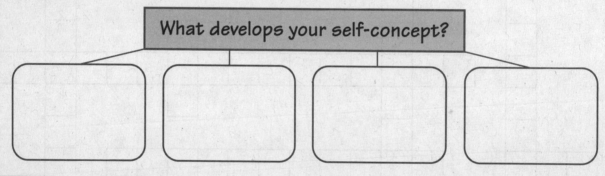

What develops your self-concept?

Lesson 2 pp. 316–319

Summary A ________________ is something that you want to achieve.

Lesson Details Read "Setting and Reaching a Goal" on page 319. Use the information to set a short-term and a long-term goal. Make plans to reach both of the goals.

Lesson 3 pp. 320–325

Summary Anger that can harm others physically or emotionally is called ______________. When you have strong feelings, you need to use ______________ when you express your feelings. Sometimes you feel ______________ when you have too much to do. When this happens, listening to music or reading can be good forms of ______________.

Lesson Details Describe some of the signs that show each kind of feeling.

aggression ______________________________

stress ______________________________

anxiety ______________________________

Lesson 4 pp. 328–330

Summary People who are about your own age are your ______________.

Pressure from them to do something is called ______________.

Lesson Details How are negative peer pressure and positive peer pressure similar? How are they different?

____

____

____

____

Lesson 5 pp. 332–335

Summary A belief that everyone in a certain group has the same characteristics is a(n)

______________. A negative attitude toward an entire group is a(n) ______________.

Lesson Details Describe how prejudice and stereotypes keep people from cooperating.

____

____

____

Lesson 6 pp. 336–338

Summary A(n) ______________ arises when people do not agree. Peacefully

solving a problem when people do not agree is called ______________.

Lesson Details Look at the chart on page 337. Describe a situation in which you could use the steps to resolve a conflict.

Name ______________________________

Focus Skill
Reading Skill

Identify Main Idea and Details

Conflicts

As you have learned, conflicts happen when people do not agree about something. Some conflicts are small—for example, a disagreement with a friend about what movie you want to see. Other conflicts are large—for example, a disagreement between two neighbors about how loud their music can be played. What is important when you are involved in any conflict is to be able to solve the problem peacefully by using the steps for conflict resolution.

When you disagree with someone, it is important to listen carefully and completely to his or her side of the situation. Knowing fully what the other person thinks can help you work with him or her to reach a resolution. When you express your own opinion on the matter, you should stay calm and speak in a respectful manner.

Once opinions have been expressed in a conflict, it is time to brainstorm possible solutions to the problem. By brainstorming together, the parties in a conflict can usually come up with a compromise that will satisfy both sides. Someone who is not directly involved in the conflict can act as a mediator and help find a resolution to the conflict.

After ideas are suggested, the parties involved in the conflict must choose the idea that will best resolve the conflict. Sometimes one person must "give in" while the other person seems to "win." It is better to think of these situations as compromises that help both parties maintain their relationship and move forward past the conflict.

Complete the graphic organizer by supplying the Main Idea and Details you learned from reading about conflicts.

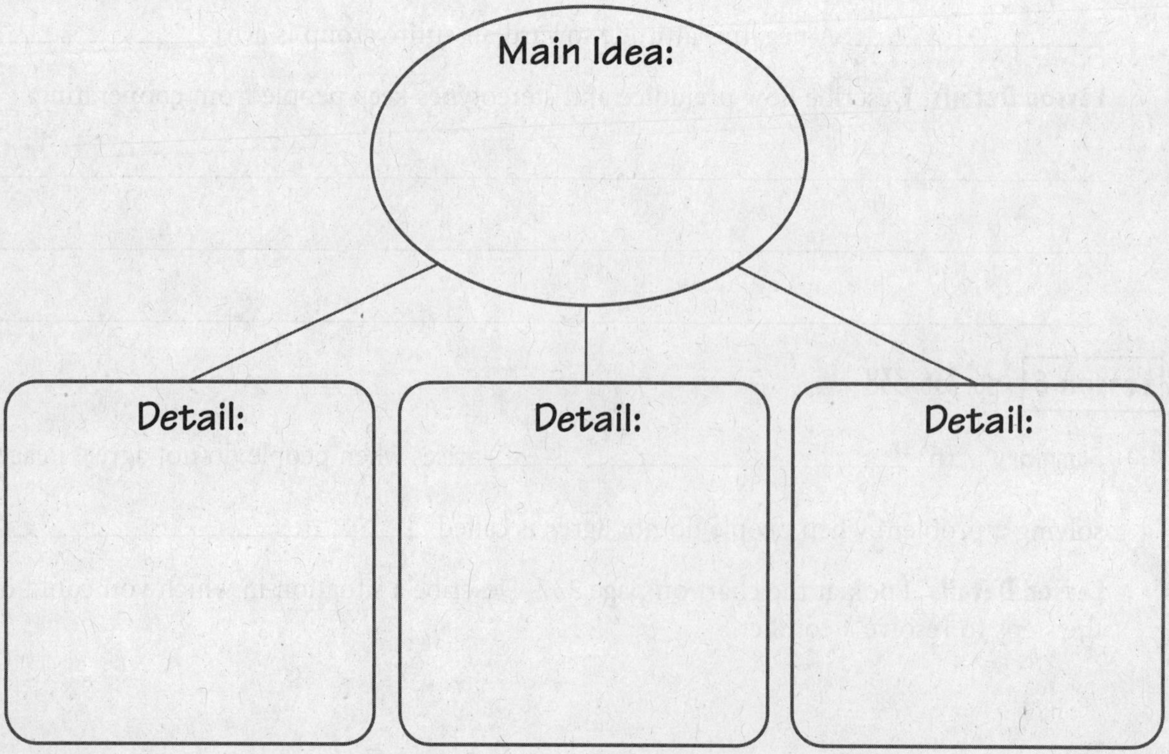

Name ______________________________

Problem Solving

Life Skill

Manage Stress

Steps for Managing Stress at School

1. Know what stress feels like.
2. Try to determine the cause of the stress.
3. Do something to relieve these feelings, such as preparing to handle the stressful situation.
4. Relax by listening to music or reading.

Tell how these students could use the steps to help manage stress.

A. Ling tried out for her first school play and was chosen to play a supporting role. After two months of rehearsals, the first show is tonight. Whenever Ling thinks about the performance, she suddenly forgets her lines and where she is supposed to stand.

- How could Ling manage the stress she feels before her first performance?

____

____

____

____

____

____

____

B. Paco has studied hard for a social studies test that he has to take in third period. However, each time he thinks about taking the test his palms get sweaty and he feels as if he has butterflies in his stomach.

- How could Paco manage the stress he is feeling about taking his social studies test?

____

____

____

____

____

____

Name ______________________________

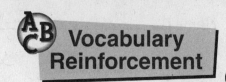

Vocabulary Reinforcement

Matching

A. Write the letter of the term in Column B next to its meaning in Column A.

Column A

____ **1.** Judgment about an entire group that is not based on fact

____ **2.** How you think of yourself

____ **3.** Belief that everyone in a group has the same characteristics

____ **4.** Painful sadness that can last for a long time

____ **5.** Properly managing your emotions

____ **6.** Something that you want to achieve, such as earning an A on a test

____ **7.** Emotional pressure that can cause physical problems

____ **8.** An uneasy feeling

____ **9.** Variety among people

____ **10.** Respect for yourself as a person

Column B

a. self-control

b. goal

c. self-concept

d. stress

e. anxiety

f. prejudice

g. grief

h. diversity

i. stereotype

j. self-respect

B. Choose two of the vocabulary words from Part A. Then write a sentence or paragraph comparing the two words.

____

____

____

____

CHAPTER 11 Name ______________________________ Quick Study

Family and Responsibility

Directions

- Use lesson vocabulary and other terms in the Word Bank to complete each **Summary**.
- Read the section directions to complete each **Lesson Details**.

Word Bank

communication	cooperation	responsible	sibling
compromise	respect	self-discipline	

Lesson 1 pp. 344–346

Summary Becoming a ______________ person is an important part of growing up. A responsible family member shows ______________ for family traditions and follows family rules. If you are responsible, you are a person who practices ______________.

Lesson Details Use information from pages 344–346 and your own experiences to correct the graphic organizer. Circle each phrase that describes a responsible family member. Cross out each phrase that does not.

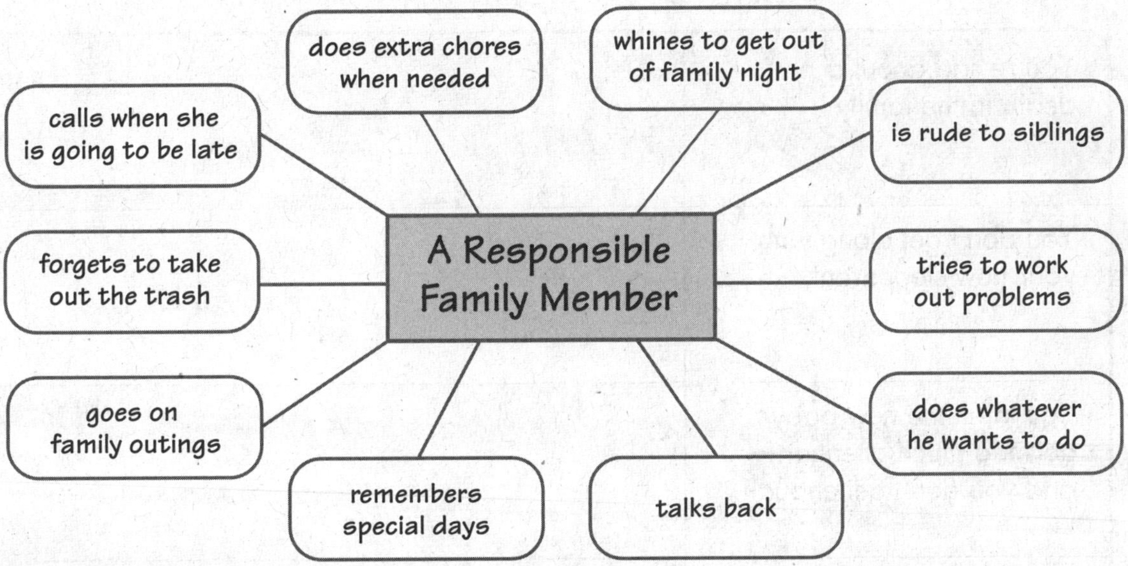

Lesson 2 pp. 348–351

Summary A successful family practices two important things: ______________ and ______________. Family members talk to each other and work together. When they disagree, they ______________ by looking for a solution that will satisfy everyone.

Name ______________________________________ **Quick Study (continued)**

Lesson Details Use the information on the clipboard on page 351 to complete the chart.

Action	Details
Talk	over problems.
Listen	
Accept	
Admit	
Be	

Lesson 3 pp. 354–358

Summary All families go through changes. Family changes include moving, illness, divorce, and getting a new ______________. Some changes may be painful. It's OKAY to ask for help.

Lesson Details Use the information on page 358 to fill in the chart. For each kind of problem, fill in at least one source you could go to for help.

You're sad about a death in the family.	
You don't get along with your new stepparent.	
You think the new baby gets too much attention—and you don't get enough.	
You've just moved to a new school, and you don't know anyone there.	

Name ______________________________

Focus Skill **Reading Skill**

Draw Conclusions

Twin Troubles

Read the paragraphs and answer the questions.

Heather's family moved to a new town last month. Heather is adjusting to her new school. She is starting to make new friends and learn her way around the neighborhood. She even joined a club at school and is planning to try out for the girls' basketball team. Heather's twin sister, Haley, is not adjusting as well. She mopes around the house in the evenings. Some mornings, she claims she is too sick to go to school. Her grades are falling. Her temper is short, and she cries and yells about the simplest things.

Heather is worried about Haley. She tries to talk to her, but Haley slams her bedroom door and tells Heather to leave her alone. Then Haley yells through the door, "Just hang out with your friends. You care more about them anyway!" Heather answers, "If you'd stop hiding in your room and come with me, we could both be happier."

1. What conclusions does Heather draw about Haley?

____

2. What conclusions does Haley draw about Heather?

____

3. What conclusions can you draw about things that Haley might do to adjust to the move? Use the graphic organizer to show your conclusion and the information you used to reach it.

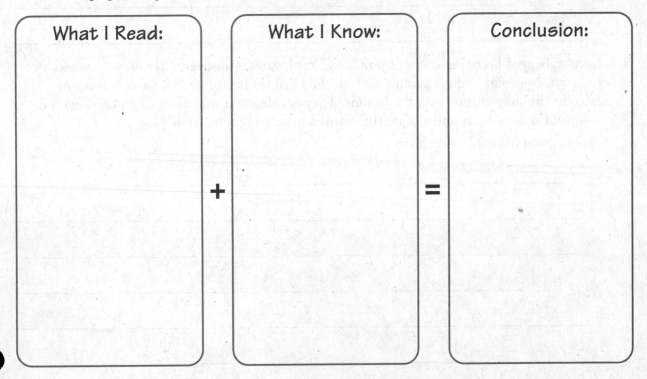

What I Read:	+	What I Know:	=	Conclusion:

Name ____________________

Problem Solving

Life Skill

Resolve Conflicts

Steps for Resolving Conflicts

1. Use "I" messages to tell how you feel.
2. Listen to the other person. Consider the other person's point of view.
3. Negotiate.
4. Compromise on a solution.

Use the steps to help these students resolve conflicts.

A. Soledad and her younger sister Maria shared a room after Maria was born five years ago. Now each girl has her own room. However, Maria keeps coming into Soledad's room and bothering her. Soledad puts a sign on the door that says "Private! Keep Out!" Maria is in tears.

- Explain each person's point of view and suggest a solution.

B. Malcolm begged his parents to let him take guitar lessons. However, after only six weeks of lessons, Malcolm told his parents that he had changed his mind. His parents thought Malcolm should continue with the lessons. They decided that Malcolm should stick with the lessons for at least six months. If he still wanted to quit then, he could.

- Is the compromise fair? Explain.

Name ______________________

Vocabulary Reinforcement

Solve the Word Puzzle

Use the clues below to complete the word puzzle.

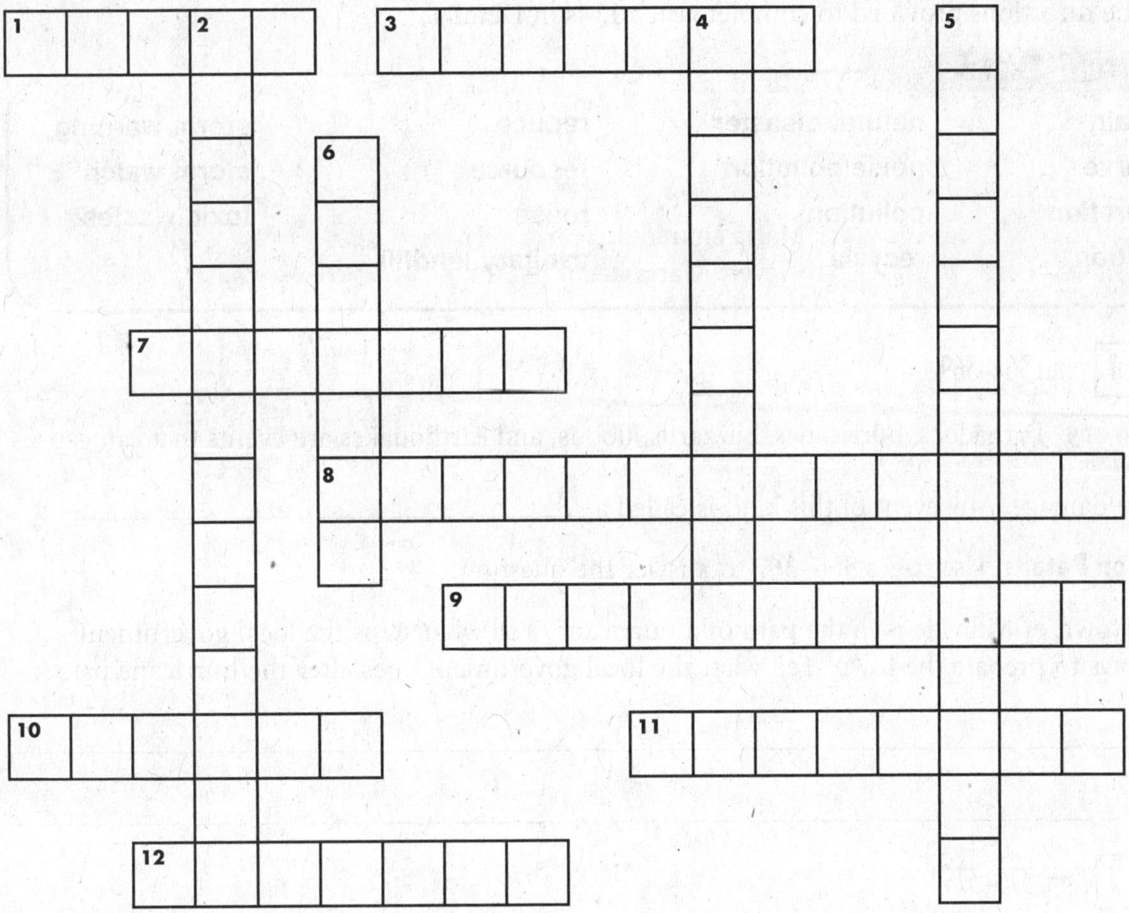

Across

1. harmful or hurtful treatment
3. appreciation or regard; seeing the value of someone
7. a brother or sister
8. talking, listening, sharing ideas and information
9. the act of working together
10. a group of related people who care about each other
11. a serious disagreement
12. to solve or settle

Down

2. the ability to control your actions
4. to settle a difference of opinion by mutual agreement
5. dependability and trustworthiness
6. the failure to take care of another person

CHAPTER 12

Name ____________________

Quick Study

Community Health

Directions

- Use lesson vocabulary and other words in the Word Bank to complete each **Summary**.
- Read the directions provided to complete each **Lesson Details**.

Word Bank

acid rain	natural disaster	reduce	storm warning
conserve	noise pollution	resource	storm watch
incineration	pollution	reuse	toxic wastes
insulation	recycle	sanitary landfill	

Lesson 1 pp. 364-369

Summary Tornadoes, hurricanes, blizzards, floods, and earthquakes are events that can cause great damage. Any event of this kind is called a ____________________.

Lesson Details Use pages 366–367 to answer the question.

The town of Millville is in the path of a hurricane. Tell what steps the local government follows to prepare the town. Tell what the local government does after the hurricane passes.

____

____

Lesson 2 pp. 370-375

Summary Weather forecasters alert the public by issuing a ____________, which indicates that a storm *may* happen, or a ____________, which means a storm is almost certain to occur.

Lesson Details Use pages 372–373 to complete the graphic organizer. Show the sequence of steps your family should follow after a severe storm warning has been issued.

1. → 2. → 3.

Lesson 3 pp. 376-379

Summary Many places dispose of trash by burying it in a large, lined hole called a ____________. In other places, trash is turned into usable electricity during a process called ____________.

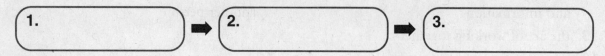

Name ______________________________

Lesson Details Use the information on page 376 to show, on a separate sheet of paper, the sequence of responsibility for ensuring food safety.

Lesson 4 pp. 380–384

Summary Any material that people use and that is obtained from the environment is called a ______________. Two resources that people must ______________ are heat energy and water. Using ______________ in homes can conserve heat energy.

Lesson Details Write *True* on the line if the statement is true or *False* if the statement is false. Use pp. 380–384 to help you figure out the answers.

______________ **1.** The Earth's supply of gas, coal, and oil is unlimited.

______________ **2.** Recycling, reusing, and reducing the amount of materials we use will conserve natural resources.

Lesson 5 pp. 386–391

Summary Natural resources must be kept free of ______________. ______________ is one type of pollution that can, over time, affect living things, stone, and metal. Waste materials, especially ______________, are poisonous to living things.

Lesson Details Use pages 386–391 to complete the sentences.

1. Most air pollution comes from ______________________________.

2. A toxic waste discarded from people's homes is ______________________________

______________________________.

Lesson 6 pp. 394–396

Summary Everyone can do three specific things to protect the environment: ______________ the number of things we use and reduce the amount of pollution we create, such as ______________. Instead of buying new things, ______________ the ones you have. ______________ materials so they can be used to make new products instead of being thrown out.

Lesson Details Use pages 394–396 to create a graphic organizer on a separate sheet of paper. Choose a product. In sequence, show steps you could use to *reduce* the amount you use, *reuse* it, and *recycle* it.

Name ______________________________

Focus Skill **Reading Skill**

Sequence

A Water Treatment Plant

Water that is to be treated so it can be used as drinking water comes either from groundwater sources (wells or springs) or from surface-water sources (rivers or lakes). Surface-water sources require a more complicated treatment process than groundwater sources. In rivers and lakes, runoff from rains causes small particles to mix with the river water. These small particles must be removed and the water made clean, or disinfected, to make it fit for people to drink.

The first step in the treatment of surface water is screening. This prevents any large objects floating down the river from entering the pumping station and damaging the equipment. The second step is a chemical pretreatment. Special chemicals destroy organisms that cause water to have a taste, an odor, or a color. In the third step, the water is disinfected by adding chlorine to it to kill any organisms that may cause disease in humans.

Next, water is mixed with a chemical that causes small particles in the water to clump together into much larger particles. This is called *coagulation* (koh•ag•yuh•LAY•shuhn). Eventually, the particles become too heavy to float and they begin to sink. Then, the water enters several large, deep tanks, where it moves very slowly. This slow-moving water allows the large, heavy particles time to settle to the bottom of the tanks. This is called *sedimentation.* In the sixth step, the settled water is filtered through a thick bed of sand and charcoal. Particles not removed in the previous step are removed here. Finally, the water is disinfected again with chlorine to kill any disease-causing organisms that might have escaped the previous steps. The water is now safe to drink.

Draw a sequence graphic organizer to show the steps used to make water safe to drink.

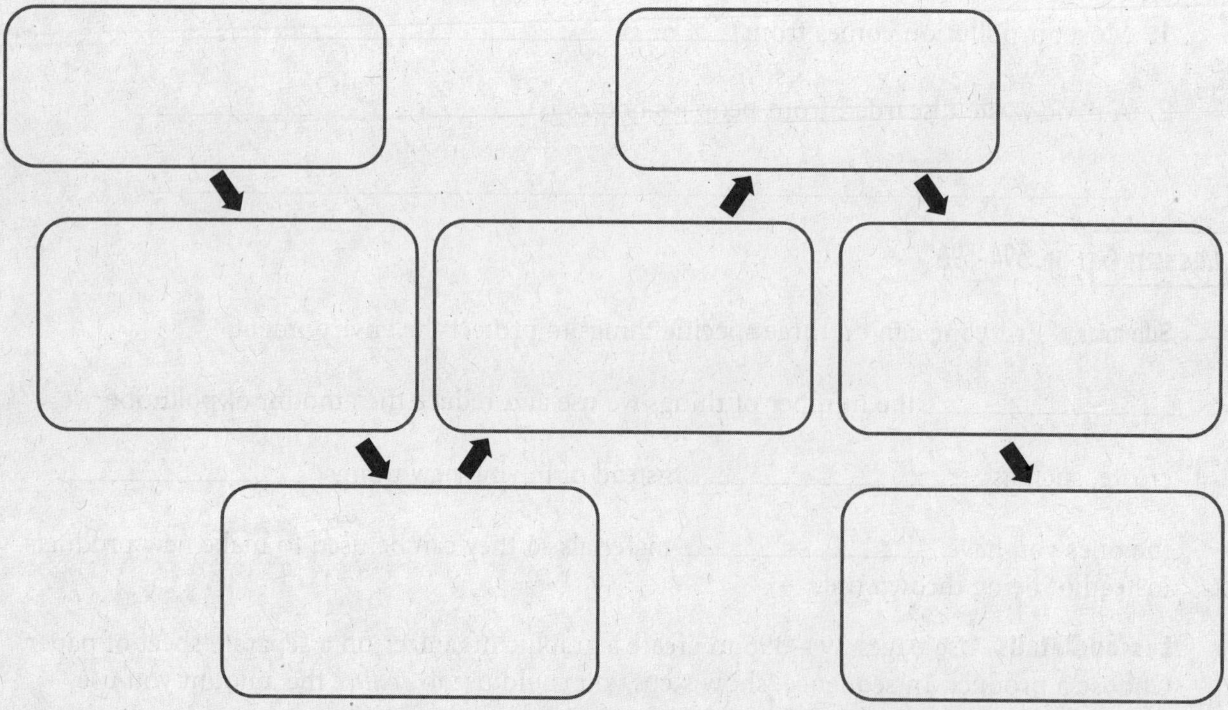

Name ___________________________________

Problem Solving

Life Skill

Set Goals

Steps for Setting Goals

1. Choose a goal.

2. Plan steps to meet the goal.

3. Check your progress as you work toward your goal.

4. Evaluate your progress toward the goal.

Use the Steps for Setting Goals to help these students reach their goals.

A. Jenna and her family just moved to California. The family members know they are living in a place where earthquakes can occur. They decide to make a family disaster plan and put together a disaster kit.

- How can Jenna and her family reach their safety goals?

____

____

____

____

____

____

____

B. Mr. Clark wants his students to participate in Save-Our-Environment Month at his school. He thinks practicing the three R's would be the best way for his students to participate. He would like his students to continue the project for the entire month.

- How can Mr. Clark use the Steps for Setting Goals to make a plan for his students?

____

____

____

____

____

____

____

Name ______________________________

Vocabulary Reinforcement

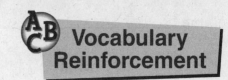

Use Word Meanings

From the box below, choose the term that best fits each definition.

a. acid rain	**e. insulation**	**i. recycle**	**m. sanitary landfill**
b. catalytic converters	**f. natural disaster**	**j. reduce**	**n. storm warning**
c. conserve	**g. noise pollution**	**k. resource**	**o. storm watch**
d. incineration	**h. pollution**	**l. reuse**	**p. toxic wastes**

____ **1.** an event in nature that causes great damage

____ **2.** a notice that severe weather *may* strike an area

____ **3.** a notice that severe weather is almost certain to strike an area

____ **4.** a large, lined hole in the ground, used for trash disposal

____ **5.** the process of burning solid waste

____ **6.** any material that is from the environment and is used by people

____ **7.** to use resources carefully

____ **8.** materials used to conserve heat energy

____ **9.** the presence of harmful materials in the environment

____ **10.** rain that damages the environment because it contains acids

____ **11.** poisonous wastes

____ **12.** devices that reduce pollution from cars and trucks

____ **13.** to improve the environment by using less

____ **14.** to improve the environment by using things more than one time

____ **15.** to conserve by reusing materials to make new products

____ **16.** loud and disturbing sounds made by human activity